Dedication

To Mary Black

To our partners and our families who support us when we get these ideas in our heads, and to all those people and alliances in the International Mental Health Network in the UK and throughout the world who have influenced and supported our work especially Piers Allott, for the inspiration to develop a workbook and Phil Thomas for his support.

Marius Romme and Sondra Escher must be specially mentioned for their work in raising the awareness of the community to hearing voices amongst well people in society and reporting widely their findings and experiences. "Accepting voices" and "Understanding voices" have been influential, setting the scene in which we could get support for this workbook. Romme has argued for a many years that hearing voices in itself is not a symptom of an illness rather the persons reaction to hearing voices can give rise to mental health problems. Romme himself said that ....." If voices are not open to cure, then they might only be open to coping". It is our belief in this statement that drives our work.

Acknowledgements

We cannot overstate the influence of many our friends in this work. Marius Romme, Sondra Escher, Paul Baker, Anne Sykes, Mike Grierson, Alan Howells, Terry McLaughlin and his family for helping Ron to get out of the system and finally but most importantly to people who hear voices and professionals who can "hear" voices.

Enduring mental illness is a failure not of individuals but of society ....for offering nothing!

Ron Coleman & Mike Smith 1997

THIS BOOK BELONGS TO
EAST GLOUCESTERSHIRE NHS TRUST
THORN COURSE

BROWNHILL CENTRE
SWINDON ROAD
CHELTENHAM   TEL 01242 275070

Preface

Professor Marius Romme, Sandra Escher

This book is a great achievement in developing a change in attitude and approach towards hearing voices.

This book is for voice hearers and the people they select to support them. It will enable people who have difficulties to cope with their voices and to discover different sides to their voices. Following a systematic approach it will unfold their relation with the voices and by doing so will stimulate them to acquire more effective ways of coping. Most important in this process, and well stimulated in this workbook, is to take ownership of the experience from writing one's own life history in relation to ones voices. Becoming more curious about the voices is stimulated by the questions and promotes ownership as well.

This book stimulates you to plan ones own life again, this is especially helpful for those who are feeling to overpowered by the voices to become their master.

In social fields and in medical care hearing voices is seen as the consequence of mental illness. Voices are felt only to be very negative, and must be controlled by professionals. Voices are hardly ever interpreted as the messengers of the persons life history.

This book however helps a person to overcome three handicaps:

1) The idea that hearing voices is the consequence of an existing illness within the person, most likely being schizophrenia, an illness of unknown origin.

2) The idea that schizophrenia is a diagnosis of an illness not related in an understandable manner with the life history of that person.

3) The idea that the person as the consequence of the illness concept is powerless against the voices, that the voices are not owned by the person, while in fact the voices are a persons own experience understandable from the personal trauma's or overpowering problems with life.

Let us first explain how Psychiatry came to look at hearing voices. It has already been 100 years since Kraeplin formulated the concept of 'illness entities' in clinical psychiatry. in this concept all symptoms are seen as the results of an existing illness within the person of which the origin is still unknown. Science in the meantime has proven that the construct of an existing illness entity is not valid. Schizophrenia for instance is a construct that represents a broad range of complaints shown by very different persons (Bentall 1990, Boyle 1990 etc. etc.).

Schizophrenia does not represent a diagnosis. in a diagnosis one tries to understand what has led up to the complaints. One analyses the complex interaction between the persons capacities, the personal development and social conditions s/he is living in.

The term schizophrenia, in the classification system as used in the DSM, represents a category based upon a rather broad range of available symptoms at a certain moment or period in time. This period does not tell us anything about the possible causes nor does it include the personal experiences and their meaning for the person involved. Neither does it indicate how to cope with the experience.

Calling a person who cannot cope with the voices 'ill' is understandable when the voices and the emotions or behaviour they provoke are dominating the persons functioning and life. It is reasonable to call the person 'ill' when the voices are not an integrated part of the person but destroy ones free will. It is not right however to look at hearing voices in itself as a symptom of an illness. No it is the coping with that experience that might give rise to the emotions and behaviour that can be called ill.

Therefore a person who hears voices but cannot cope with them, needs support to overcome the powerlessness and to be able to begin living again. Support is needed in coping with voices, Support is also needed in order to become stronger in ones own identity. Lastly support is needed in accepting that what has happened has happened and should not be felt guilty about rather it needs to be placed back in the life history, placing the responsibility where it belongs with the activist not the recipient.

It is the great merit of Ron Coleman that he has seen these three handicaps in his own life and with great persistence has changed his life. Becoming a victor after having been a victim. He did not deny what has happened to him, but became critical in a way that made it possible to build his own life. His second great merit is that he found companions in the mental health professional world.

It is the vision of Mike Smith that has seen the value of Rons' work and has joined with him to follow this different road. They wrote in partnership this fantastic book. It is a great opportunity that Mike and Ron have worked together to develop this practical support system for those voice hearers who intend to build up their own life. Not denying the hard work to come but commencing on the road instead of waiting for some coming wonder. This book is based upon our research as far as overcoming the first handicap is concerned, It is based on Rons' private experience as far as the second and third handicaps are concerned. It is however further based upon the experience of many other voice hearers met in support groups in the UK. These people have taught Mike and Ron to ask the right questions. it is based on experience, not yet on scientific evaluation.

Romme & Escher 1997

Introduction

We decided to write this workbook in response to both users and professionals asking for some written material on how to work with voices.

Ron Coleman

After much reading I came to the conclusion that most of what was written was written in jargon and restricted hearing voices to the clinical framework. This means that many voice hearers are kept in the dark by the use of clinical language. A friend of ours, Sharon Le Ferve when talking about self harm talks about self harm as an intermediate language. Reading her book "Killing Me Softly" makes me think that there must be an intermediate language in other areas of mental health, especially in psychosis, which can easily be likened to a language.

From many professionals the language heard is the language of illness, of the hopelessness of the chronic patient. For users this translates into the language of apathy, fear, despair and sometimes into actions such as self harm or even suicide.

I too believe in a language. It is the language of fighting back of liberty of victory, it is the moving away from being a victim to becoming a victor. I no longer believe in allowing people to empower me in small things, I believe in taking power in all things.

This workbook is about stopping being a victim of our experience and becoming the victor over our experience. It is not meant as all things to all people, rather it should be seen as a starting point for exploring our experience. It contains no magic cures only hard work that hopefully will challenge us to move forward. We spend many hours talking about the changes that we need to make in our lives to get our act together, but we must ask ourselves how many hours do we spend making the changes.

Ron Coleman 1997

New Eras for professionals?

Discussion in the development of social and democratic psychiatry in the latter part of the 20th century commonly refers to the need for a 'paradigm shift'. This is seen as a prerequisite for any significant alteration in the values and style of the way in which support is organised and provided for people in mental distress.

A paradigm shift simply means the change in fundamental beliefs about something that alters the way we see the world. Paradigm shifts as conceptual realities were introduced by Kuhn who spoke of the beginnings of all revolutionary changes being heralded by a break with the old ways....... to interpret our worlds differently based upon a new way of thinking.

This argument pervades most discussions yet the paradigm shift is often portrayed as a holy grail mythical in appearance and elusive in reality. I often wonder if that elusiveness is convenient and that in order to have a paradigm shift you would need to have a commitment to see the world differently and it is that commitment, not the opportunity that is missing. Seeing the world differently relies upon new information it is the evidence and personal experience of the phenomenological approach that the hearing voices movement brings that has offered me a different frame of reference for mental distress. I know this is shared by many other colleagues.

Marius Romme in an unpublished paper writes-

"When a paradigm has been proven not to be scientifically valid it is not wise to keep on practising and researching as if the paradigm was valid. But the trouble for professionals is what to do otherwise." Marius further postulates that professionals are blinded by their training and the use of the illness model. This leads them to view all symptoms as part of an illness of unknown origin even though the symptoms may be a reaction to situations that lead to "illness" Because of this we are unable to look at the new world with our traditional paradigms

The opportunity is with us in that new approaches are available to professionals that totally depart from the most fundamental approaches of psychiatry to date, and these approaches have been with us for a number of years yet little is being done to develop approaches that reflect an alliance rather than a dispute with service users.

The long awaited paradigm shift will be evident if professionals accept what users have been telling them for a long time and that the victor to victim workbooks try to capitalise upon. This is that their experiences are real and that only by working within a conceptual framework which accepts those experiences as real can any positive strategy be developed by the person to move from victim to victor. Only the person can become the victor. Our jobs should be to help them on the road from victim to victor. I hope working with this book helps professionals and voice hearers to begin to see the world differently. I have been and am still, struggling to throw off the veils that my training has given me. I hope this workbook can help others to try new systems of working and to evaluate their experiences doing so.

Challenging the psychiatric orthodoxy?

Working within traditional frameworks if you are not yet ready for a move, no matter how much biomedical research and social research tells us of the reasons for voices it rarely offers ways of working with the voices. Perhaps the only unifying factor in most research is agreement that the person is experiencing something which in some incidences is distressing.

Most traditional methods of dealing with voices either

a)   Treat voices as symptoms of illness

b)   Deny the voices

c)   Deny the experience

Although limited these approaches appear to have worked for some people.

A further approach that has and is being tried is to accept the voices by understanding them and accepting them as part of their lives. This is an effective alternative for some people and perhaps most significant is in evidence in a high proportion of those people labelled as severely mentally ill who consider themselves to have recovered.

This work is all about the tool kit. It is not a cure all as there are no magic cures; however, we do realise that there are opportunities for users and professionals to actually for the first time in our experiences to make alliances. These alliances to work together have begun to emerge from people who are prepared to listen, to hear the voices and to support the person to develop their ways of constructing their lives to incorporate all their experiences and to live their lives.

We are not talking here of any rocket science. This is not the realms of eminent people, it is about human behaviour that has been socialised out of us in our western culture to support our friends in their time of need, and to butt out when they no longer need us.

Empowerment is the language of professionals. It is passive it gives power, power is not given it is taken. Myself and Ron do not believe in empowerment we believe in liberty and emancipation. We hope that this workbook can help some people to take control and regain their liberty.

We have worked together in an alliance. We do not lie to each other that we have the same agendas. We do not and we will not. What we have is common ground and we meet on the common ground. I hope that other people will meet on the common ground and will try to work within the realms of the person who hears voices, not to try to enforce them into the realms of the professions.

Mike Smith 1997

What are the origins of this workbook?

Firstly the hearing voices movement has been central rather than insidious. It has been predominantly led by voice hearers themselves and because of the nature of the discussions has tended to be beyond non voice hearers. This movement is above value and it would be negative to try to replace it ,or even worse to professionalise its approach. Rather, there may be a role for friends and professionals to use the known ways of coping to develop joint strategies with people to enable them to live with voices.

Following the work, most notably of Romme & Escher but also the UK experiences of Paul Baker and others, hearing voices began to be seen as not the exclusive prerogative of saints and psychotics. Although this is by no means a widely accepted theoretical approach, rather it was found that a lot of people who are apparently not mentally ill heard voices. By looking at the experiences of both groups of people it was hoped to develop strategies for voice hearers to accept the voices.

It is important if you are going to commence this work, or share this work with another person, that you agree ground rules. I would suggest that you follow these rules.

Ground rules for working together

1   The person who owns the experience owns this workbook. If it is decided to make any paid person or friend aware of some of its content then it must be with acceptance of the ground rules.

2   The person needs to develop their own ways of coping with voices. Any support should reflect the persons own experience and definitions not the person supporting them.

3   The experience is real.

4   Trust is not implicit, it is earned. Every professional has broken that trust. Every service user has had trust broken innumerable times bear this in mind. Every time a person asks for trust they give of themselves and every time it is broken that part of them is killed. You pave the way not just for yourselves but for other well meaning people who may follow.

5   It is all right for new coping strategies to be slow to work. Many people try different ways of dealing with the voices. It is better to try and partially succeed than to never to try at all. You are in charge as long as you try. You are no longer the victim you are now the victor.

The Workbook layout

This workbook is organised to reflect the intentions outlined. It is for either a voice hearer to use or for them and a friend or paid supporter to use together to see if there is a common ground upon which they can work.

Take breaks regularly, there are no time limits, you dictate the pace. You don't have to complete the book. You may find some parts more useful than others.

Part one

Understanding voices is for you, and with your permission a chosen person, to *understand and contextualise* your experiences. This may be the first time you have explored your experiences This can be hard both for you and the person who is working with you to travel new ground. We hope it can completely change the way you and others around you see your experiences. **Pg 11-20**

Part two

Is about how you currently *organise your experiences*, what they are and how they affect you. **Pg 22-33**

Part three

Is about *accepting and working with the voices* and developing strategies for you to take control. **Pg 34-50**

Ownership

The workbook remains the property of the person who hears the voices. It is personal and, if shared, is confidential. If you are a professional or friend then simply giving this workbook to someone offers them an alternative. If they choose to use it with you then you can use it as the common ground where you meet, and can identify what support they want from you to enable them to recover, in their way, from this experience.

Developing an action plan to deal with your experience

Most professionals are required to plan and record what they do for you. You can use this to help you, if you choose, when working with professionals. This plan should be focused around **your** experiences and how **you** understand them, and should work to your goals and nobody else's. The basis for most plans is some form of appraisal. There is no reason why this should not focus around you and your voice hearing experience. We give a guide at the end of this book for you and your chosen supporter to use the work done in this book, as a base to identify your own plan of action.

We have both found great positive results from working with— not against voices. Voice hearers have found that they are not alone, that others have become victors and that by identifying their own experiences they can try to organise their experiences in such a way that they can begin living again, but living with the voices.

An important message

We cannot, and do not stress enough in this book that this work is ongoing and hard and at first you may not find the coping strategies immediately working.

It's okay when things don't work !!!

They will in the long run, if not directly, by giving you the energy to look at the way you see the voices and understand them. From this you can try new ways and think of your own by moving from the **victim to the victor.** We are always pleased to hear from people who have used the workbook and include an evaluation form at the back for this purpose. If you can find time to give us your comments and experiences it can help us when we edit this workbook or develop further ones.

Understanding your experiences

The onset of voices

When the voice hearing experience begins there can be a multitude of responses. The very first reaction is at an emotional level whether this be positive or negative. It is not surprising that such a personal experience involves what can be the extremes of emotion. Romme and Escher describe the onset of voices as the startling phase. The first time I heard a voice I was sitting at my desk waiting for some information from the computer when a voice behind me said " you've done that wrong". I looked around thinking it was my secretary but there was no one there. My first feeling was fear. My response was to go to the bar and get drunk.

It is important that you can look back to your first experience of voices. Below there is room to write a description of your first experience of hearing voices. Include everything you can remember. It is all right to be honest. You don't have to share this with anyone you do not want to. This can be a stressful thing to do, but write as much as you can, even if it doesn't seem important now. Many people have told us how just writing these things down make them feel better about them.

Response

....

....

....

....

....

....

....

....

....

....

Now that you have written up your first experience read it again, and make sure you have not missed anything, no matter how small. If you have, add it now.

....

....

....

If not, let's move on to Accepting voices

Whether you have just recently started hearing voices or if you are exploring old voices for the first time, the starting point remains the same, and that is to accept the reality of your voice hearing experience. Answer the following question.

Are your voices real to you ?   Yes   No

If your voices are real to you then here is some good news, *you are not alone,* in fact you are in very good company. Many great people throughout history have heard voices, these include, Moses, Jesus, Mohammed, Socrates, Joan of Arc, Swedenbourg, Bruno (the philosopher), Jung, Churchill, Ghandi and more recently Anthony Hopkins, Zoe Wannamaker and Micheal Barrymore. For many of the above, the voices they heard were an inspiration and although this is not always the case, it is useful to remember that it does not always have to be painful.

Your initial response may decide how you feel about your voices, so please answer the next questions.

(i)   Do your voices frighten you ?   Yes   No   Sometimes

(ii)   Do your voices make you angry?   Yes   No   Sometimes

(iii)   Do you realise you may have   Yes   No
        positive voices?

(iv)   Do your voices invoke any other strong feelings?

....

....

....

It is not surprising if your voices frighten or make you angry. Many voice hearers have described the onset of voices as sudden, startling and a period of great anxiety. They experience the voices as both negative and aggressive from the very beginning.

This type of encounter with voices makes it difficult to accept the experience as a normal occurrence. It leaves many with their lives in chaos and isolated from family, friends and society. Many voice hearers feel forced to withdraw completely from society into themselves, where they only relate to their voices and may become overwhelmed.

It is important that you acknowledge how you respond to the voices. On the next page describe your responses to voices. Do not worry if you think other people will find them strange. It is your experience, not theirs, that is meaningful.

How did you respond to your voices ? Describe your feelings, actions and anything else you consider useful. With this section Take your time!! Take breaks!! Stay cool.

....

....

....

....

....

....

....

....

....

....

....

....

....

Read again what you have just written. Is there anything you can learn about yourself from it ? When I did this exercise for myself I learned a great deal about myself, the most important thing being how I attempted to deny what was happening to me. It was this denial at an early stage that I now believe meant I spent so many years in mental distress. Write below anything you can learn about yourself about how you have responded initially or in the past to your voices.

....

....

....

....

Have you or other people tried to deny what is happening to you telling you that you are wrong, if so write down who.

....

....

....

If so how did this make you feel? It can be very annoying to be told you are mad or constantly wrong. Write down how you felt.

....

....

....

Has anybody helped you or listened? If "yes" these can be strong allies in your recovery. Name them below.

....

....

....

....

Life History

Romme and Eschers' research revealed many things but one of the most important was that 70% of those they interviewed started hearing voices after what Romme and Escher called a traumatic life event. These events included death of a loved one, (normally violent e.g.. suicide or murder or accident) leaving home for the first time, abuse be it sexual, physical or emotional and being involved in a major disaster are but a few of the life experiences that voice hearers disclosed in their interviews with Romme and Escher.

Sondra Escher has expressed on many occasions her belief that one of the most important things that a voice hearer can do is to write what she calls their ego document. An ego document is a persons life history written by themselves and more importantly, for themselves. *The writing of your life history is the single most important thing a voice hearer can do for themselves.* Through writing your life history in your own style you can bring out what is important to you. It is an opportunity to move away from how others view your life and what has happened to you in it. We all have a story to tell about our lives, no two of which are the same. It is important that you start to see your self as an individual rooted in society and not as a patient rooted in psychiatry.

On the next four pages write your life history in a condensed form. If there is not enough room then use separate sheets and insert them into this workbook. Use your own language and keep it simple. Do not try to analyse as you are writing just be factual. Remember, this is for you, so you can be as honest as you like. You need never show the contents to anyone.

LIFE HISTORY BY.......................

Response

....

....

....

....

....

....

....

....

....

....

....

....

....

....

....

....

....

....

....

LIFE HISTORY BY.........................

Response

....

....

....

....

....

....

....

....

....

....

....

....

....

....

....

....

....

....

....

LIFE HISTORY BY..........................

Response

"I've just heard voices" checklist

Now complete these next two pages each time you hear voices for the next 10 days at least. Feel free to photocopy these two pages.

Date .... Time spent with voices ....

Time .... Voluntary time with voices ....

Please be as honest as possible as this checklist is to help you identify the voices, and any things which occur that can help you to identify when the voices communicate with you, and to develop ways of predicting and organising your life to accommodate the voices.

The voices I heard were:-

1 .... 4 ....

2 .... 5 ....

3 .... 6 ....

The voices said

....
....
....
....

They were talking about

....
....
....
....

I Felt

....
....
....
....

I Was at (Place)

....
....
....
....

I Was with (Company)

....
....
....
....

I was doing

....
....
....
....

The place was (Noisy, quiet, people talking)

....
....
....
....

I had been thinking about

....
....
....
....

Please answer yes or no

My state of consciousness was altered   _____

My Vision was heightened/altered   _____

I felt Paranoid   _____

I felt out of control   _____

I felt powerful   _____

My explanation for the voices is

....
....
....
....
....
....

Please add any other information that will help you develop your work either alone or with people

Organising your Experience

Frames of reference and relationships with your voices

If you accept the reality of your voices experience, and have carried out all the excercises, you have probably moved into what Romme and Escher call the organisational phase. Put simply, the organisational phase is when voice hearers attempt to understand their experience by explaining for themselves where their voices come from. This stage is also about building relationships with your voices. This is sometimes called finding a frame of reference. Frames of reference vary from person to person and some people have more than one frame of reference.

What is a frame of reference?

A frame of reference is the process of explaining your experience within your own belief system. Everyone has their own belief system about their voices. Your belief system is as valid as anyone else's; indeed, you know better than any of the people paid to 'help' you. Use the rest of this page to write about what, who, or how you believe the voices are. What do they mean to you?

Response

....

....

....

....

....

....

....

....

....

....

....

The most common beliefs about voices given by voice hearers are as follows:-

1 : Illness

2 : Psychological

3 : Telepathy

4 : Spiritual

5 : Demons or the Devil

6 : Angels, Saints or God

7 : Technological

8 : Aliens

Please take your time to write down your beliefs about your voices. If you agree with the above say so and write about it. If you have other beliefs write them down.

....

....

....

....

....

....

....

....

....

....

....

....

Belief Systems

You have written down your beliefs and understanding of your experiences. We will now look in detail at some common belief systems, medical, psychological and telepathic. You may find it useful to explore these belief systems yourself in order to clarify for yourself your beliefs. From this you can begin to understand your current ways of coping and how you relate with your voices.

The Illness Model

Many people believe that voices are a symptom of mental illness. Voices are considered a first rank symptom of various mental illnesses such as schizophrenia, manic depression, affective disorders and some types of depressive illnesses. The majority of people who hear voices are treated for what is called a psychotic illness and the main type of treatment is the use of neuroleptic medication. Neuroleptics are drugs which work by inhibiting the chemical dopamine which is a naturally occurring chemical found in the brain. The effect of the neuroleptic medication is to reduce or remove the voices, thereby allowing the person to get on with their life. The above is a simplified version of the theory behind the medical model for most, though not all, psychotic illnesses.

If you believe in the illness model for voices then you will probably be on, or have been on, one of the following drugs: chlorpromazine, stelazine, haloperidol, sulpiride, modecate, depixol, clozaril, or rispiradone. These are the main major tranquillisers, though there are many others in use which are in the main derivatives of those mentioned above. Below write all the drugs you have been on for your illness.

Drug name	What were you told that the drug was for?	What effects did you notice?
....	....	....
....	....	....
....	....	....
....	....	....
....	....	....
....	....	....
....	....	....

Did the drugs get rid of your voices ?   YES   NO

If no, did they reduce the voices ?   YES   NO

If you have answered "yes" to any of the two previous questions above then write below which drug or combination of drugs worked for you.

Response ....

....

....

One more question you should ask

Do you feel you have the same quality of life now as you had before you started hearing voices?

Response ....

....

....

If you have answered that your life is back to normal then get on with it, although there may still be some mileage in reading further. If, however, you feel your life is not back to where it was, or where you want it to be, then read on.

Side Effects

For many people the side effects of the medication they are on are often described as worse than the illness being treated. Many others find that they must endure these side effects in order to have any kind of life at all. Is this how you view your life on medication?

YES   NO   SOMETIMES

If it is, then you may have a problem getting on with a normal life. All the evidence available, such as the study carried out by Donaghue, suggests that the more information you have about the side effects of medication then the better you will cope with the side effects. Do you know all the side effects of your medication?

YES   NO

24

If the answer is "no" then there are a few things you can do to find out. By far the easiest is to ask your CPN, if you have one. They should have books which list all the drugs and their side effects. If this is not an option ask your local chemist or find a book on medication at your library. There should be some in the reference section. Your local MIND association or advocacy group should also be able to help. It will be useful if you write down the side effects you have. Use the space below to do this.

The side effects I have are

....

....

....

....

There are many other forms of "treatments" available within a medical framework. Please write down which you know you have tried and the effects they have had on you, good and bad.

....

....

....

....

....

Have you ever been offered any form of therapy or talking treatments? If "yes" describe their effects if "no" write down what you think may, if anything, help in talking treatments for you.

....

....

....

....

....

....

Facts and Fiction in the illness model

A great deal of fiction surrounds the illness model and voices. Unfortunately much of the fiction dished up as fact comes from professionals. Much of it is based upon making generalisations from a very small research base. Let us look at some of the facts and fictions surrounding what psychiatry calls auditory hallucinations.

Fiction : Hearing voices is a symptom of schizophrenia.

Fact : 80% of people who hear voices are diagnosed schizophrenic. Hearing voices is also a part of many other mental health problems and found in the mentally well.

Fiction : Medication cures people who hear voices.

Fact : There is no evidence that medication cures. What it can do for some people is to suppress the symptoms. This is not a cure, rather, it is symptom management.

Fiction : In schizophrenia medication is the treatment choice for hearing voices.

Fact : We know that medication works for 33% of people this is the agreed recovery rate from illnesses such as schizophrenia.

Fiction : Medication is the only effective treatment for people who hear voices.

Fact : Up to 50% of people with a diagnosis of schizophrenia still hear voices when treated with medication.

Fact : Dr William Sargent presented a paper in 1966 entitled " The Recovery Rate In Schizophrenia Prior To The Introduction Of Neuroleptics." The research covered the period up to 1938 and Sargent showed that the recovery rate in 1938 was 33%.

Fiction : Psychotics cannot be treated using talking treatments.

Fact : There is evidence to show that talking treatments can be effective in working with people who hear voices. However, the number of talking treatments has never been significantly explored, nor is this frequently offered as an alternative for people who hear voices.

As you can see there are many views about the "facts" presented about the medical model about voices, but let's not throw out the baby with the bath water. If you are one of the 33% who recover; then there is no point in jeopardising your recovery by stopping your medication. If, however, you still feel that the illness model offers you no relief then perhaps it is time to explore other frames of reference. You can do this on your own but it would be easier if you did it with someone else.

A word of caution— *stopping* your medication is not a wise thing to do without medical advice as the sudden cessation can cause a tardive psychosis, which for many is worse than the reason they were put on the medication in the first place.

The Psychological Model

The term psychological model may sound a real mouthful and difficult to understand, and if we were to continue in this type of jargonistic language you would find it difficult to understand this section. .

For some the psychological model will conjure up the need for clinical psychologists to be intervening with some form of therapy. For myself the term psychological means much more, and does not mean that you have to have professionals involved in your recovery, though you may wish to do so.

When we talk about the psychological model what we mean is that you believe that the voices come from within yourself, and are rooted in a life event, normally an unpleasant one which may have happened many years before. If you look at your life history you may be able to pin point life events which you feel are at the root of your voices. It may help if you write below any of the life events that you think may be the cause of your voices.

Life events (use your life history as a guide) that are significant to my voices

....

....

....

....

....

How are the above linked to your voices?

....

....

....

....

....

....

....

For myself I found two major life events that I believed were the root of my voices. They were: being sexually abused as a young boy and the death by suicide of my first partner. Such events are not uncommon and people respond in different ways to them. In recent times people who respond by hearing voices are sometimes diagnosed as having post traumatic stress disorder, though in the past schizophrenia was a much more likely diagnoses. It is important that you work through what you think about your diagnoses (if any). Answer the next two questions. If you do not know the answer to question one then ask your GP or CPN. If they are unable to answer ask your psychiatrist. If she or he is unable to give you a diagnosis (some do not feel it is helpful) then write and ask what you are currently being treated for.

What is your diagnosis?

....

....

Do you agree with your diagnosis?   YES   NO   DON'T KNOW

If you are in the system and you disagree with your diagnoses and further, you voice your disagreement, then you are probably described as a non compliant patient or you will have been told that you lack insight. If this is the case then it is important that you work through what is happening in a systematic way. One of the ways of doing this is to start by looking at your voices in detail. This can be a difficult exercise and it may be useful to carry it out with the help of someone you trust.

Do you agree with your treatment?   YES   NO   DON'T KNOW

When answering the following questions take your time and think through your answer Feel free to make more comments on the page marked notes at the end of the questions. Remember you do not need to show this to anyone if you do not want to.

How many voices do you hear?   ....

How many of your voices are male?   ....

How many of your voices are female?   ....

Are any of your voices positive?   YES   NO   SOMETIMES

If yes or sometimes how many?   ....

Are any of your voices negative?   YES   NO   SOMETIMES

If yes or sometimes how many?   ....

Are any of your voices advisory?   YES   NO   SOMETIMES

If yes or sometimes how many? ....

Are any of your voices commanding?   YES   NO   SOMETIMES

If yes or sometimes how many? ....

Are any of your voices abusive?   YES   NO   SOMETIMES

If yes or sometimes how many? ....

If you know the names or if you have given names to any of your voices, then list them below please feel free to comment on your voices here.

Response

....

....

....

....

....

....

....

....

....

....

Now, to start to identify your voices and to record them so that you can begin to establish who the voices are, when you hear them, and any other relevant details. Please photocopy this list on the next two pages and fill one each time you hear the voice(s). Try to complete it as soon as possible afterwards and try to carry on your normal life whilst doing this. Do not listen for the voices any more than you normally do.

From the questions you have just answered and the voices checklist you have completed it is possible to build up a voices profile for each voice. Below you will find descriptions of three of the voices I hear, not as I hear them now, but how I heard them in the early days. The three voices are called Priest who was my abuser Annabelle who was my partner who died and Neil, a close friend who also died. One of the things you should notice is the difference in personalities between the voices.

Name	Male/Female	Pos/Neg	Advisory/Command	Abusive
Priest	Male	Negative	Commanding	Yes
Annabelle	Female	Both	Both	Both
Neil	Male	Positive	Advisory	No

Using the rest of this sheet do the same for the voices you hear. If you cannot name all the voices you may find it useful to describe them in some way e.g., you may think the voice reminds you of a teacher so call it Teacher, or you may think a voice is a demon so call it Demon.

Name	Male	Pos/Neg	Advisory/Command	Abusive
....	....	....	....	....
....	....	....	....	....
....	....	....	....	....
....	....	....	....	....
....	....	....	....	....
....	....	....	....	....

If you wish to add anything more about the characteristics of your voices, or need more space to finish your voices profile, then use this space.

Response

....

....

....

....

Now that you have carried out the voice profile it is time to make decisions about how to move forward. Start by trying to relate your life history to your voices profile. If you can relate any bits of your life or events to your voice profile then write them below.

Response

....

....

....

....

....

....

....

....

How would you like to work with your voices? Are there things you have identified at this stage about your voices that can help you to work with them?

....

....

....

....

....

....

There are many other wide frames of reference (social, genetic, spiritual, cultural) that we do not have time to go into, rather, we will look at one of the more specific frames of reference as a working example to approaches of working within your framework.

We will now look at a very specific belief system that is commonly held as one example. There are however many others. We will look at how you may work (with support if you prefer) with telepathic voices.

Telepathy

Many voice hearers believe that their voices are due to telepathy; that is, they believe that they hear other peoples thoughts. This can be extremely distressing and startling for voice hearers, and this distress is often compounded and amplified disproportionately by the attitudes of families and professionals, which is normally to deny the experience (see the ground rules), to prescribe or increase medication, or to look to residential support for the voice hearer.

The reason for all this is the non acceptance of the person's belief system, which leaves the professional in effect as helpless as the voice hearer. They have no tools to help from without of their own beliefs, hence the cosy coercion toward the professionals system of reference.

If you believe your voices have a telepathic component try asking a professional or person who you are close to fill in the following.

I .... believe that telepathy and my sensitivity to it is one reason for the voices I hear, please describe in as honest a way as possible your response to me.

....

....

....

....

....

....

No doubt there will be conflicting opinions. This conflict is not useful for either party in working with voices.

There is, however, another way of working through this experience. The starting point is something that has been repeated time and time again in this workbook, and that is acceptance of the experience. If both parties accept the realities of the experience then we can start developing a coping technique within the voice hearers understanding of what is going on. There are two ways of looking at Telepathy, one is as a psychic phenomenon the other is to give it a psychological frame, i.e. that the person is very sensitive to others, their feelings etc. (it is interesting to note that even within a psychic framework telepaths are often referred to as sensitive and open to others).

In order to work within a persons frame of reference it is necessary to accept the former explanation that the voice hearer is indeed experiencing some form of telepathic communication.

By validating the persons experience it is then possible to work together to resolve the distress caused by the experience. Again being systematic is the key to success. It may be useful to start by both of you reading books around the psychic experience such as "psychic self defence". Some may find this difficult, especially if they have been taught to think that it is impossible to work in what is called a delusionary framework without colluding, but doing nothing has not succeeded, so lets give it a try. For example, say the person who is hearing the voices hears voices that tell them to kill themselves, then I would ask the person to ask the voices why, and to give them a reason. You do not let voices get away with answers like "you deserve it" or "your evil". You need a proper explanation Remember you have the right to say no!!!!!!!

Please record your experiences

....

....

....

Even within telepathic explanations it is possible to achieve peace when you need it. Here is a exercise that requires practice until you perfect it but once you do, you should be able to relax when you wish. If your belief system is telepathy then you are basically saying you have a gift. If this is the case then you more than likely have other gifts. One of these will probably be the ability to block out negative thoughts that you are receiving by building a psychic block. The easiest way to do this would be to pick a point in front of you and in your mind build a wall that will not let negative thoughts through. It may take you some time to get it right but it will be worth it.

Please record your experiences

....

....

....

....

....

Telepathy is then like any other explanation for voices. All you need to get through it is the ability to work through the experience, looking always for positive ways to resolve difficulties.

33

Accepting and Beginning to Live with Voices

Coping Strategies

Coping strategies which are used by voice hearers are often described as maladaptive, that is, they are seen as not being of any real benefit to the voice hearer. For example in the work of Nick Tarrier and others telepathy is described as a maladaptive framework that should not be encouraged This is despite the fact that a great many voice hearers use telepathy as their explanation for what is happening to them.

Coping strategies can only be understood by understanding the belief system of the voice hearer. This then is the leap that many professionals fail to make. The failure is not theirs, rather, it is a product of their training.

This section is an introduction to coping strategies which voice hearers use with varying degrees of success. It is impossible to predict which of the following strategies will work for an individual and even harder to list the number of strategies available. It is important that you try different strategies until you find the one(s) that work for you **START SMALL!!!**

Like most voice hearers you will have probably already developed some coping techniques of your own. You may not even have realised this ,but do not worry. It is normal for people to adapt to what is happening to them.

Romme and Escher in their book " Accepting Voices " divide coping strategies into three types :

1 : **Cognitive Strategies**
   Which include, ignoring the voices, listening to the voices, listening to the voices in a selective way, telling the voices to go away and getting into a meaningful discussion with the voices.

2 : **Behavioural Strategies**
   Which include, distraction techniques, (e.g., activities), negotiating with the voices keeping a diary. meditation

3 : **Physiological**
   Which include, alcohol, drugs, medication, relaxation and diet.

These lists are in no way exhaustive and only show the diversity of coping techniques. It may be that you already use one of the above methods or perhaps you have one of your own.

Below write down any coping techniques that you use and state how well they work for you.

....

....

....

....

....

....

You may find that you have done little to date formally with your voices. that's okay, you done well surviving so far, most people we know have felt powerless at times, gaining power is a slow process it is more important that you find the path that is right for yourself than blindly following others.

....

....

....

What would you like to change, if anything about your voices and how you respond to them?

....

....

....

....

....

Let us now turn to developing strategies that may help you work within different frames of reference (or ways of thinking). The more approaches you try the greater your opportunity of finding a system of reference that will help you to recover.
The following are not all the ways in which you can work with your voices. You may have developed your own that is successful to you. If so, all we seek to offer are additional tools to help.

Your ways of working with voices

It is important that you write answers to each of the questions in as much detail as you can. Come back to questions if you are unsure, or if you want to add to them later. This profile of your experiences we feel, should be central to any plan you develop to work with your voices. You need to try ways of working recording your experiences. If you have a plan of support with a professional then this workbook can help you both to ensure that any support you can get is geared around your way of working.

What other things have you tried that have worked (including help from others)?

....

....

....

....

....

....

What help would you have liked to have been offered?

....

....

....

....

....

What if anything can professionals offer to you?

....

....

....

....

....

How would you like this help ? When & Where?

....

....

....

....

....

....

....

Who should do what?

....

....

....

....

Is their anything that you would not like to happen to you if you are suffering from the effects of the voices?

....

....

....

....

....

....

We can only offer as alternatives what friends and colleagues have given us of their successes and toils working with voices, and our own experiences.

Understanding Voices

If, after the work you have done you are able to answer the following questions it could help you to develop a strategy to understand and work with the voices so that you are able to organise your life with them.

Do you know the reasons for your voices?

....

....

....

....

Do you know why the voices communicate with you?

....

....

....

....

Do you know what they mean to you?

....

....

....

....

....

Exploring

Throughout the next few pages remember think small steps don't be too ambitious.

Have you spent time exploring the voices not just listening to what they say?

....

....

....

Do you know how to work with them for your benefit, to take some control?

....

....

....

Have you explored if any of the voices are related to your life events?

....

....

....

Have you explored ways of dealing with the feelings you have from these events?

....

....

....

Have you tried negotiating with the voices? If not why not?

....

....

....

Are any of your voices reasonable?

....

....

....

Do you have any allies in your voices?

....

....

....

You need to build your strengths from your alliances with the positive voices .
Are there times when they are reasonable?

....

....

....

Can you refuse to listen to the voices until they are reasonable? have you tried it?

....

....

....

Structuring time

Have you set time aside to work with the voices ?

....

....

Have you set times to listen to the voices?

....

....

Please describe how you have tried and what is successful to organising time spent with the voice (s)

....

....

....

....

Tuning in

Are there positive voices you want to work with?

....

....

Positive voices can have positive outcomes. Can you use one voice to help you with the ones that you do not want to listen to?

....

....

Can you focus upon one voice? Can you be selective?

....

....

Can you exclude other voices by focusing on one?

....

....

How do you do this?

....

....

....

....

Allowing/Disallowing

Some people find it helpful to practise allowing the positive voices to speak above the negative. By negotiating, you can agree times for this. As well as this you can try disallowing the voices you don't want by tuning in to the positive messages and using the voices that support you. Try this and record the results. Don't worry if it doesn't work, it takes practise and perseverance and good understanding support to do this.

....

....

....

....

Working Paradoxically

People have told us that they can summon the voices at times that they find convenient, this then allows them to schedule times when the voices will leave them alone and when it will be important not to be distracted for instance in a job interview or going out with your friends. If you feel confident you can try this however if you are one of those people for whom any break is a relief or you are afraid of the voices then take your time, small steps at a time is a good thing to remember. Write down your attempts.

....

....

....

....

....

....

Physical methods

It is surprising how effective for many people physical exercise can be a first way of both coping and living. One method that is practical and is easily practised is vigorous walking. If you are having a dialogue with your voices in a public place then walking quickly is a good way of doing this and not standing around for long keeps you out of harms way. The effects of physical exercise on the body is well known, its effects on the mind to a lesser degree. There are seemingly limitless ways of being physically active, try ones that suit you, keep a record of any results.

....

....

....

....

....

....

Developing a strategy to work voices

Hearing voices as a survival strategy. Hearing voices can be legitimately seen as a survival strategy. Indeed one of the main points of this workbook is to accept and work with the voice. If removal of the voice is your aim then fine, but don't let anyone talk you into believing that to recover the voices must go. This is not true; many members of the community hear voices The voices you hear may help you to survive. Do you think you are able to cope with the events you wrote of in your life history because of the voices?

please tick   Yes   No

If "yes" then you should not aim for the voices to go completely. You need to aim to organise them so that they do not significantly affect you until you feel you want and are ready for them to go.

If "No" then you can aim for the voices to be organised in such a way that they are of little relevance to you.

What do you do as a result of the voices? Do you speak with them, argue, fight, laugh with them, agree, disagree etc.

....

....

....

....

After reading the work you have done in the workbook you may have some clearer ideas of how you intend to work with your voices.

If you would like to involve people who are paid to help you in this plan, I would suggest you use the following format.

Beginnings/ working with professionals

Many people will have discussed assessments and other forms that they have to fill in with you. It is the way that professionals base and justify their plans. If you wish to own the process of recovery (which we feel, and others have done, is critical for emancipation) you may want to place yourself at the centre of the planning process. This is so that the plan will follow your needs, wishes and wants rather than focusing upon problems and beliefs defined by other people without reference to you. To make the most of the resources that are available to help you, you need to make professionals work with you and your voices not fighting to get you to deny them.

You need to be able to tell the person you want to work with some of your coping strategies and the way that you want them to work to support you in working with the voices.

If you have a life history in this book you may wish to disclose elements of this to any meetings. Write down beforehand those things about you feel it is important that people know and also the conditions in which you wish them to be known i.e. that people don't tell other people about them. Write down who you do not wish to know.

Planning

You should, if possible, attend a planning meeting with someone you can trust who is aware of what you want. Plan it beforehand. If you don't wish to involve a friend or partner ask for the addresses of your local advocacy service.

Write down what you want from services. There is no need to be specific. Take this as a list to the meeting and be clear that the plan is for you, not to make life easier for the services. Be honest. (if you feel having a job is important say it.).

What I want in my plan:-

....

....

....

....

Identify your voices that are a concern for you. Look at your coping mechanisms. What are they?

      voice/name   how I work with it

1
2
3

What else do I need to support me with the above mechanisms?

....

....

....

....

Who should do this?

....

....

What choices do I have available from working with this book that I haven't tried?

....

....

What groups of people with similar experiences are there that I can get help from?

....

....

This workbook is necessarily limited. We know that there are many other areas we should cover but cannot in these pages, rather, we aim to offer you alternative views . We hope you have learned that there is a process of liberation and you must work through and own this process yourself, with help at your direction. Use the principles of understanding, organising and accepting your voices to help you to start living again.

The A-Z of coping with Voices

Accept the reality of your voices

Break through the victim barrier

Consider all your options

Develop coping strategies that suit you

Enter into dialogue with your voices

Focus in on your voices

Go to a self help group (a hearing voices group if their is one)

Help others by sharing your experience

Identify the areas of your life that you need to work on

Join in activities outside of mental health organisations

Keep a diary

Live your life not your label

Make space for yourself

Negotiate with your voices

Own your voices

Perseverance is the name of the game

Question your voices

Reward yourself when you succeed

Small is beautiful

Take your time haste can mean failure

Use services to your advantage

Victories have to be fought for

Work on your weaknesses

Xperiment with different coping strategies

You make your decisions not your voices

Zap your negative voices by gaining control over them.

Memorandum of agreement

Coping strategies can only be understood by understanding the belief system of the voice hearer this then is the leap that many professionals fail to make. The failure is not theirs' rather it is a product of their training. So can we work through our experience to a successful resolution without the involvement of professionals especially if they refuse to work within our frames of reference? The answer to this is yes but it is much harder as we will always be in conflict about the way forward.

It is in both parties interest then to negotiate a way of working together that may require compromise but as long as the compromise is on both sides then it is the basis of a working relationship.

It may be useful then to write an agreement between yourself and the professional/ person you are working with write your agreement below then sign and date it.

The following is the agreement made between   Name
and   Name

This agreement determines how we shall work together with my voices

Signed

Signed

Remember that you are the centre of this process, it is there to support not disable you. You have a right to expect good service.

Treatment wishes of ....

To whom it may concern I .... being of sound mind this date.......................... would like to record that in the event of me being treated without my informed consent would like the following to be considered and adhered to as is my expectation of my civil rights.

I do not want the following treatments to be given to me.

Please list (some people list ECT, medication,)

I would like the following approaches to be considered as a priority and my wishes (people list, leave me alone, let me lie in bed, listen when I speak to you, listen to my experiences, maintain my respect and dignity as a person)

Please contact the following people in event of my admission to hospital whom I would like to be involved as my representative.

Name
Address

Telephone

Please note that the following person is the person whom I would like to act as my representative above my legally defined next of kin.

Name
Address

Telephone

The solicitors authorised to act on my behalf in matters concerning my mental health and liberty are

Name
address

Telephone

(If desired)

To my key worker ....

Please record this information in my case notes/ care plan/ records. As my paid professional support I expect you to act with my interests uppermost .

I .... (key worker) recognise the wishes of .... and agree that I will always endeavour to act in their interests and to make people aware of these choices in treatment pathways.

Evaluation

We hope you have benefited from working with this workbook. Remember that recovery is a process, the ends are difficult to achieve, most people consider themselves to be recovering not to have recovered.

If you would like to comment on this work book we really would like to hear from you positive and negative. Please write your comments on this form, tear this out and return it to the address below. Further copies are also available from this address.

....

....

....

....

....

....

....

....

....

....

....

....

....

....

....

Please return to
Mike smith
C/0 Handsell publications
136, Crow lane West
Newton le Willows
Merseyside
WA12 9YL

NOTES

NOTES